Strategize Meals To Boost Balance Diet And Health

Get rid of fat, live healthily and fit, expand lifespan and increase metabolism.

Elizabeth C. Palmer

DISCLAIMER

scanned, faxed, or retained without approval from the publisher or creator.

Table of Contents

Introduction

Chapter 1
Understanding Metabolism and Nutrition

Identifying Factors that Influence Metabolism and Ignite Fat Burning

Chapter 2
How to Balance Macronutrients and Incorporate a Variety Of Foods to Optimize Nutrition and Support Weight Loss

Chapter 3
Unveiling Effective Strategies for Timing Meals and Snacks to Maximize Fat Burning and Metabolic Efficiency

Cycling into Success: Exploring the Impact of Calorie cycling on Metabolism and Long-Term Weight Management

Chapter 4
Enhancing Metabolic health with Functional Foods: Harnessing the power of functional foods to boost

metabolism, support fat loss, and improve overall health.

Identifying key superfoods and their specific benefits for metabolic function and longevity.

Chapter 5
Exploring Different Types of Exercise and Their Effects on Metabolism

Exploring Different Types of Exercise and Their Effects on Metabolism

Chapter 6
Sustainable Strategies for Long-Term Success

Conclusion

Introduction

With the help of this revolutionary guide, we will go on a journey towards complete nutritional wellness and energy. I will investigate the intricate connection between health benefits, the body's metabolism and general healthy living.

In this world of rapid change, achieving and sustaining the best possible health may seem like an unattainable goal when you're trying to achieve it. Trying to figure out how to achieve actual wellness can be difficult because of the prevalence of foods that are processed, the prevalence of popular diets, and the inconsistent tips that are given regarding diets. But there is no need to be concerned because this book will act as your guide, a beacon that will show you the road to a life that is healthier and full of vitality.

At its essence, this book revolves around advancement; at its most fundamental, it empowers you to take charge of your health, shift how you deal with food, and reveal the keys to mastering your metabolism. You will be equipped with the expertise and tools needed to thrive by delving into the fundamentals of dietary intake, metabolic processes, and healthier living habits. This can be accomplished by utilizing a blend of studies supported by scientific evidence, practical techniques, and everyday life instances of achievement.

However, this book is not just about eliminating excess weight or reducing one's outfit size to an appropriate one. There are a great many other aspects to consider. A balanced strategy to well-being that goes far beyond the number that appears on the scale is what it means to nourish the body from within outwards, to power your metabolism with foods rich in nutrients, and to embrace an all-encompassing approach to wellness. It's about experiencing your best life full of force, vigor, and happiness.

In this book, you'll discover the life-changing impact of tactical meal planning, a tailored strategy for dietary needs that incorporates your particular metabolic demands, health objectives and lifestyle decisions. From regulating calories and scheduling meals for maximum energy to introducing micronutrients and nutritious foods that enhance your metabolic system, each chapter is filled with helpful recommendations and realistic techniques that aid your success.

But presumably, the most significant aspect of this book addresses sustainability, creating routines and conduct that contribute to long-term health and vitality. We'll cover the significance of consciousness in consuming food, discovering pleasure in activity, and establishing a supportive atmosphere that allows you to stay on track regardless of what difficulties may come.

So, if you want to reduce persistent pounds, enhance your energy, or embrace a healthier, fuller life, this ebook is your guide to success. It's time to quit the diet beliefs, achieve your health, and adopt a lifestyle that provides nourishment to your body, boosts your metabolism and raises your general well-being.

Are you ready to begin this transforming path toward optimal health and energy? If yes, let's explore together and uncover the potency of planning meals to unveil the path to metabolic control and lifetime wellness.

powerhouse, a key to that petroleum products our every motion, thought, and breath. Welcome to the realm of metabolism, where an intricate ballet of molecules regulates the musical score of life itself.

Envision the following: your body is a full metropolis, with trillions of cells full like busy commuters, with each having its mission for keeping a metropolitan area running smoothly. At the core of this lively cityscape lies metabolism, a multifaceted system of biochemical processes that transform food into energy, govern key activities, and support life.

But what precisely is metabolism, and for what reason does it matter?

Metabolism, simply described, is the sum of every single chemical response that takes place within your body to sustain life. It's the process by which your body turns the food you eat into the vitality it requires to power everything from respiration to participating in races. Imagine it as your body's greatest multitasker, a tireless worker who never tunes off.

Chapter 1

Understanding Metabolism and Nutrition

In the immense maze of the human body, there resides a silent workings of this metabolic masterpiece.

Envision your body as a sports-performance car, regularly in need of fuel to keep its engine churning. This energy source comes in the form of food carbohydrates, fats, proteins, and even alcohol all of which supply the raw elements and energy your body needs to function.

But here's where it gets interesting: not all foods are created equal if it comes to feeding your metabolic engine. Just like a high-performance automobile runs better on premium fuel, your body flourishes when fed by nutrient-dense, entire foods filled with minerals, vitamins, and radicals.

Carbohydrates, for instance, are the body's main source of fuel, delivering the fast energy required for racing through your day. Nevertheless, not every carbohydrate is made equal opt for complex carbohydrates like vegetables, fruits, and whole grains, which deliver constant power without the jolt and burn of processed sweets.

Proteins, on the other hand, are the fundamental elements of life, vital for healing tissues, developing muscle mass, and controlling metabolism. Incorporating lean sources of protein like chicken, fish, soybeans, and beans into your daily diet can help keep your metabolic flames burning strong.

Furthermore, let's keep in mind the overlooked outstanding individuals in the nutrition world. While fats have earned a poor image in previous years, they play an essential role in the production of hormones, brain functioning, and food digestion. Aim for wholesome fats like fruit such as avocados, almonds, seeds, and olive oil to keep your body's metabolism whirring over effectively.

But here's the twist: Your metabolism isn't solely dependent on the food that you eat, it's also controlled by a variety of factors that range from genetic factors and age to hormones and exercise level. You must look at nutrition with a comprehensive mentality, taking into consideration not just the foods you eat, but how you consume how much you eat, and even how you exercise your body's needs.

Consider your metabolism as a beautifully tuned instrument, delicately balanced and receptive to the symphony of messages it gets from your environment. By knowing the foundations of metabolism and its complicated interplay with dietary habits, you possess the pathway of unleashing your physical being's full potential for well-being, energy, and lifespan.

You may assume your metabolism, whether rapid or sluggish, is something you're born with, passed down from your parents. Some folks do seem like they've been born with a strong metabolism and can eat anything they want without gaining an ounce. But there are various things that you can manage that affect your metabolism and your weight.

Anabolism in comparison to catabolism

Metabolism is split down into two processes: anabolism and catabolism. Anabolism is the conserving of energy, sustaining new cells, and preserving body tissues. Catabolism is the reverse, breaking down energy to produce motion, heat, and fuel your body.

Basal Metabolic Rate?

Your initial metabolic rate (BMR) is the number of calories you require to keep your metabolism functioning when you're resting. Your BMR offers your body the energy it needs for several essential functions that are going on all the time, without you knowing about it. For example, you need it to: Breathe air into your lungs, Pump your blood Break down your meals, and, develop and heal Make and

manage your hormone levels
Keep your body warm

People can have varying BMRs. About 60%-70% of the energy your body utilizes goes toward your BMR. But your BMR may vary based on: Health Create and manage your hormone levels

Keep your whole body warm. People may have varying BMRs. About 60%-70% of the energy your body utilizes goes toward your BMR. But your BMR may vary based on: The extent to which muscle you have, How much fat you have, how old you are, how many calories you eat how active you are

Some people think your sex plays a role, although at least one study didn't discover it to have any impact on BMR. Exercise might also influence your BMR, but it's not simple to detect how. If you need to relax a lot, it may go down. If you run a lot and then stop, even that may cause your BMR to fall. Your BMR also can fluctuate for plenty of causes that scientists and doctors don't understand. Your BMR can also alter. For example, if you try to lose weight and limit calories severely, it will make your BMR go down. That's why it can look like you'll lose weight fast at first and then you'll observe weight loss slow down.

Blaming weight-related issues on metabolism is a simple task. Keeping one's weight stable, on the other hand, is a complicated process which entails several factors, including the body's hormone diet, lifestyle, naps, workouts, and stress.

A sluggish metabolism is the result of a combination of inactivity and a reduced requirement for energy. For example, when you offer your body an excessive amount of energy in the form of calories, that energy will be stored as fat since it has nowhere else to go.

To keep your weight stable, your metabolism is working hard. It is not possible to make significant modifications to your daily routine after only a few days of doing so.

Your metabolic system will be able to recognise a new optimal weight if you maintain a balance of healthy practices.

You are the director of your metabolic ensemble, and with the appropriate information and nutrition, you can put together a composition of health and well-being that will resonate for a lifetime. Therefore, as you embark on this road of exploration and metabolic mastery, keep this in mind: you are the band leader of your Increase metabolic ensemble.

Identifying Factors that Influence Metabolism and Ignite Fat Burning

Consider your metabolism to be a thriving business, with nourishment being purchased, sold, and traded in an endless cycle of energy exchange. However, as in any business, the distribution of goods and services can be driven by a variety of circumstances, each of which plays a distinct function in molding your body's metabolism.

1. Genetic factors

Our biological makeup, like the pack of cards shuffled at birth, serves as the basis for our metabolic path. A number of us are born with a rapid metabolism that appears to readily burn calories and melt fat. Certain individuals nevertheless, may be dealt a less favorable hand, with genes that incline them to slow metabolism and persistent fat storage. You cannot modify your genetics, but you can optimize your surroundings and habits for metabolic performance. Knowledge of your genetic code allows you to play the hand you're dealt by adopting healthy habits and optimizing your surroundings for metabolic success. Understanding your inherited traits and attempting to deal with them, instead of fighting them, can help you achieve long-term fat loss and metabolic balance.

the complicated movement of gene expression, the intricate waltz that determines which genes are activated and deactivated in response to environmental stimuli. While your genetic code may serve as a framework for your metabolism, the interaction of genes and the environment ultimately decides your body's ability to burn fat. Certain lifestyle variables, such as nutrition, exercise, and stress, can all alter gene expression, promoting or inhibiting fat burning. Making strategic decisions that support healthy gene expression, such as consuming a highly nutritious diet, committing to consistent exercise, and effectively managing stress, can help you shift the metabolic switch and open your body's full fat-burning potential.

In the age of customized healthcare, genetic examination is known as an effective instrument for deciphering the complexities of our DNA and gaining insights into our metabolic health. By analyzing important metabolic genetic traits, researchers can find potential inherited traits that may affect your body's capacity to burn fat and respond to certain lifestyle treatments. Equipped with this knowledge, you may adapt your diet, exercise, and other lifestyle choices to better match your genetic composition and maximize your burning calorie capacity. Genetic testing can provide significant information that allows you to take charge of your metabolic fate, whether it's altering your macronutrient ratios, modifying your workout programme, or introducing tailored supplements.

2. Age is the waiting time for weapons

As the years pass, so does the ticking time bomb of retirement, wreaking havoc on your metabolism with each new birthday candle. As we get older, our rate of metabolism naturally slows down due to a variety of reasons such as decreasing muscle tissue, fluctuating hormones, and adjustments to our lifestyles. But don't worry with the correct tactics, you can defy the ageing process and maintain your metabolic fires burning bright long into your elderly years.

3. Hormones, the Chemical Messengers

Hormones are chemical signals that govern bodily processes. They are one of the causes of being overweight. The growth hormones adiponectin and the hormone insulin, as well as male hormones and growth hormones, all have an impact on our hunger, metabolism (the rate at which our bodies burn calories for energy), and fat distribution. Obese people have elevated amounts of these hormones, which promote improper metabolism and fat storage.

Hormones are the quiet puppet masters who control your metabolism from behind the scenes. These chemical messengers, which range from insulin and cortisol to thyroid hormones and sex hormones, play critical roles in controlling hunger, energy expenditure, fat storage, and muscle growth. You can achieve long-term weight loss and metabolic harmony by balancing the hormones in your body through correct eating, sleep, and managing your stress.

4. Nutrition as Energy for Fire

When it comes to fueling flames of fat loss, nourishment is the most ideal fuel for your metabolic furnace. Choose nutrient-dense, whole foods high in antioxidants, vitamins, and minerals to boost your metabolism and prepare your body for optimal performance. To keep your metabolism working smoothly and efficiently, eat lean meats, complex carbs, healthy fats, and plenty of vegetable and fruit consumption.

The three macronutrients carbohydrates, proteins, and fats are central to nutrition, with each performing a distinct role in feeding your metabolic engine and maintaining general health. Carbohydrates are the body's major source of energy, supplying the fuel required to conduct everything from cognitive function to vigorous physical activity. Proteins, on the other hand, are the fundamental building blocks of life, necessary for tissue repair, muscle development, and metabolism regulation. And don't forget about fats, among the nutritional world's misunderstood heroes who play important roles in hormone production, brain function, and nutrient absorption.

By optimizing your intake of macronutrients and selecting high-quality sources, you can improve your metabolism and prepare your body for optimal performance. Consume full, nutritious foods such as fruits, vegetables, lean meats, whole-grain products, and beneficial fats to fuel your metabolic furnace and promote fat loss.

5. Physical Activity: Progress It Or Give up

Ah, the wonderful melody of movement, the ultimate remedy for a slow metabolism. Whether you're working out at the gym, going for a jog, or simply taking the stairs instead of the lift, physical exercise is essential for speeding up your metabolic engine and sparking a fat-burning flame. Aim for a combination of strength training, cardiovascular activity, and flexibility work to keep your metabolism running smoothly and burning fat efficiently.

6. Getting enough sleep, the Unacknowledged Hero

In today's fast-paced world, napping is frequently given up on the altar of productivity and performance. But make no mistake: skipping sleep is a guaranteed method to damage your metabolism and make your fat-burning efforts ineffective. Strive for a minimum of seven to nine hours of quality sleep per night to balance your hormones, promote recuperation and repair, and preserve optimal metabolic activity.

7. Stress, The Silent Saboteur

Last but not least, we have the quiet saboteur lurking in the shadows: stress. Chronic stress, whether from work obligations, money issues, or personal problems, can wreak havoc on your metabolism, causing a cascade of chemical imbalances that encourage fat storage and undermine fat burning. To keep your metabolic mojo in control, take time to unwind and de-stress through activities like yoga, mindfulness, or simply taking a walk outside.

One of these aspects contributes significantly to your body's ability to burn fat and reach maximum health. Knowing how each of these elements relate to and affect each other can help you unlock the keys to long-term fat loss and achieve the slim, toned figure you've frequently desired. So, equip yourself with knowledge, fuel your body with the correct meals, get with meaning, and appreciate the power of rest and anxiety management to maximize your body's fat-burning capacity.

Chapter 2

How to Balance Macronutrients and Incorporate a Variety Of Foods to Optimize Nutrition and Support Weight Loss

In the fast-paced nutrition market, organizing meals is the foundation of success and a comprehensive roadmap that guides your culinary journey to optimal health and metabolic mastery. But, with so many dietary fads, contradicting guidance, and nutritional noise cluttering the scene, how can you traverse the jungle of meal planning to construct a plan that is truly tailored to your specific requirements and objectives? connect with me as we go into the heart of meal planning, learning how to create your ideal meal plan to promote fat reduction, improve health, and fuel your metabolic fire.

1. Know Thyself: Identifying Your Priorities and Specific Objectives

Before deciding on any gastronomic expedition, it is critical to first understand your metabolic profile, health requirements, and personal objectives. Do you want to lose weight, gain muscle, or simply maintain your present state of health? Do you have any dietary limitations or allergies to foods that need to be addressed? By assessing your specific needs and goals, you can build the groundwork for a food plan that is completely suited to you.

2. Evaluate Your Existing Routines: A Review of Your Dietary Landscape Next, examine your present eating patterns and dietary landscape. How does a normal day of eating look for you? Are you consuming enough fruits

and vegetables? Are you relying too much on packaged goods and sugary snacks? A thorough review of your existing eating patterns can reveal areas for improvement and lay the framework for a healthier, more balanced meal plan.

3. Established Realistic Goals: Map Out Your Culinary Journey

With a firm awareness of your requirements and habits, it's

essential to develop SMART goals specific, measured, achievable, relevant, and time-bound to help you succeed in your culinary journey. Setting specific goals, whether they are to lose weight, increase energy, or simply eat more thoughtfully, will help you stay focused and motivated while you build your ideal meal plan.

4. Create Your Culinary Canvas: Building a Plate with Purpose

Now comes the fun part: designing your culinary painting and purposefully assembling your meal. Begin by including a variety of colorful fruits and vegetables to deliver a broad range of vitamins, minerals, and antioxidants. Next, add protein from lean sources such as chicken, fish, tofu, or lentils to help with muscle growth and repair. Finally, include healthy fats, nutritious grains, and other nutritious foods in your meal to deliver long-lasting energy and keep you content.

5. Plan: Setting Up for Success

As the proverb goes, "failing to plan is planning to fail," and this is especially true when it comes to meal planning. Take the time and effort to plan and prepare your meals and snacks ahead of time, whether that means batch cooking a week's worth of meals on Sunday or prepping individual items to make mealtime easier. When struck with hunger, having healthy, easy options on hand will make you less likely to turn to harmful convenience meals.

6. Stay Adaptable: Embracing the Ebb and Flow of Dietary Life.

Last but not least, keep your meal plan flexible and adaptable to modifications in your timetable, tastes, and ambitions. Life is packed with unforeseen occurrences, and your dietary regimen should be flexible enough to accommodate the ups and downs of your life. If food or recipe does not work for you, don't be scared to substitute something else that better meets your demands and tastes.

Organizing meals serves as the conductor of your nutritional path towards maximum health and metabolic mastery. Understanding your unique needs and goals, reviewing your current habits, and creating wise goals will allow you to create a meal plan that is suited to your own needs and tastes. So, grab your spoon and kitchen apron and prepare to embark on a culinary journey that will nourish your body, stimulate your rate of metabolism, and boost your burning calories ability.

Within the dynamic fabric of nutrition, macronutrients are the fundamental components of health and energy, three potent ingredients that energize our bodies, provide nourishment to our living tissues, and operate our metabolic processes. But how can you sort through the circular path of macronutrients to design an eating strategy that is balanced, fulfilling, and supportive of your weight reduction goals when there is so much contradictory advice and dietary orthodoxy all over the place? Come along with us as we explore the art of plate balance to maximize nutrition and fuel-burning calorie success as we take you on an expedition into the core of macronutrient knowledge.

1. The Major Three: An Understanding of Macronutrients
The big three are fats, carbohydrates, and proteins. Let's

take a few moments to familiarize ourselves with them before getting into the specifics of macronutrient balancing. Your system uses carbohydrates as its main energy source to power various bodily functions, including mental and physical activities. Conversely, proteins are the fundamental units of life; they are needed for metabolism regulation, muscle growth, and tissue repair. Not to mention lipids, the unsung heroes of nutrition, which are essential for the production of hormones, cognitive function, and nutritional intake.

Ideally, you can make sure that your body possesses the energy it needs to perform at its best, support tissue development and repair, and maintain metabolic balance throughout the day by including a balance of all three macronutrients in your meals and snacks.

2. The Art of Equilibrium: Crafting a Plate That Suits Your Needs

The art of balance, a complex ballet of proportions that guarantees you're getting the correct combination of carbs, fats, and proteins to support your health and weight loss objectives, is the foundation of mastering macronutrients. Create balanced, filling meals that are full of nutrient-dense foods compared to vilifying any one macronutrient or adhering to strict dietary guidelines.

To enhance general health and vigor, start by packing half of your tray with colorful fruits and vegetables. These foods include a variety of vitamins, minerals, and antioxidants. To help muscle development and repair, add a palm-sized quantity of lean protein, such as fish, poultry, tofu, or lentils. To ensure that your meal is balanced and leaves you feeling full, finish it off with a dish of healthy fats like avocado, almonds, seeds, or olive oil.

3. Conscientious Consumption: Understanding Your Body's Cues

It's much too simple to idly stuff food into our mouths in our quick-paced, hectic society and ignore our bodies signals of hunger and fullness. However, you can have a better understanding of your feeling full and satisfied levels and make better choices regarding what, when, and how much to eat by engaging in mindful eating practices and paying attention to the signals that your body sends.

Use a few minutes to personally check in with yourself as you grasp for that next bite. Are you eating because you're bored, stressed, or just out of habit, or are you really hungry? Do you eat until you're full, or are you undereating? It is possible to cultivate a more instinctive connection with food and arrive at decisions that help you achieve good health and weight-loss objectives by reducing down, appreciating each morsel of food, and paying attention to your body's cues.

4. Selecting Rich in vitamins and minerals Foods: Prioritising Value Over The amount Standards are equally as important as volume particularly when it comes to macronutrients. Give priority to nutritional value by selecting whole, less refined meals that are high in nutrients such as vitamins, minerals, and antioxidants, as

opposed to calorie tracking or macronutrient ratios. Select complex carbs, such as those found in vegetables, fruits, and whole grain products, as they offer long-lasting energy and fiber to promote intestinal health. Select lean proteins that are high in necessary amino acids that are needed to help muscles develop and regenerate, such as fish, poultry, tofu, and lentils. Furthermore, keep in mind that foods high in beneficial fats, such as avocado, almonds, seeds, and olive oil in particular, offer vital fatty acids that assist the generation of hormones and cognitive function.

You can guarantee that you are providing your body with the essential nutrients it requires to survive and aid your efforts to lose weight by concentrating on the quality of the food choices you make rather than simply the quantity of food you consume throughout the day.

5. Adaptability and diversity are the keys to maintaining interest in the situation.

 However, surely not least, ensure to embrace adaptability and diversity in how you plan your meals to keep things fresh and avoid weariness or exhaustion. Instead of adhering to the same meals daily, explore diverse tastes, culinary styles, and methods of preparation to keep your gustatory systems active and your palette satisfied.

Explore fresh recipes, delve into various culinary styles, and engage with new ingredients to keep your meals fresh, fascinating, and pleasurable. By embracing adaptability and diversity in your meal planning, you can ensure that eating properly never seems like a hassle and stay inspired to adhere to your weight-loss and health objectives for the long haul.

In the magnificent harmony of nutrition, macronutrients stand as the major participants, powering the functions of our bodies, hydrating our cells, and directing our metabolic apparatus. By acquiring the art of macronutrients balancing and designing meals that are stable, tasty, and full of foods rich in nutrients, you can optimize your nutrition, aid your goals for losing weight, and uncover the path to a thinner, healthier you. So, take your plate and tools, and get ready to go on a culinary experience that will feed your body, boost your metabolism, and fire your calorie-burning capacity.

Chapter 3

Unveiling Effective Strategies for Timing Meals and Snacks to Maximize Fat Burning and Metabolic Efficiency

In our fast-paced society of today, it's easy to forget how important time is in the pursuit of weight reduction and metabolic mastery. However, when it pertains to fuelling your body for fat reduction and optimizing metabolic efficiency, timing is essential. Join us on a journey into the heart of strategic eating, where we'll reveal the secrets of scheduling meals and snacks to maximize fat burning, maintain the metabolism, and discover the essence of long-term weight reduction effectiveness.

1. The Impact of Meal Scheduling: Time is All things

At the heart of strategic feeding is meal timing, a deliberate strategy regarding when you eat that might have a significant impact on your body's capacity to break down fat and manage metabolism. By properly timing out your meals and snacks all through the day, you can keep your metabolic furnace running and avoid energy dumps and appetites that can sabotage your shed-pound attempts.

Opt for a variety of snacks and main meals scheduled between three and four hours apart, beginning with an adequate breakfast to boost your rate of metabolism and power your day. Then, attempt to eat fewer, more nutritious snacks and meals all through the day to keep your vitality steady and your metabolism running smoothly.

2. Morning meal, The Metabolic Kick off

Breakfast is widely regarded as the most essential meal of the day, and with good reason. Eating an adequate breakfast within an hour or two of waking can boost your metabolism, control appetite hormones, and lay the groundwork for nutritious eating patterns across the day. Aim for a combination of carbs, proteins, and healthy fats to give long-lasting energy and keep you satiated until the subsequent meal or snack.

Choose meals full of nutrients such as eggs, Greek yogurt, muesli, and fruit to give a balance of protein, fiber, and vitamins to help with metabolic wellness and weight loss. Keep in mind to stay hydrated drinking water or a herbal beverage with your breakfast can aid with digestion and keep you feeling energized and alert.

3. Meal Duration: Discovering Your Sweet Spot

When it boils down to dietary intensity, no one solution is ideal for everyone. Others thrive on three major meals each day, whereas other individuals prefer lower, more frequent meals and snacks to maintain energy levels and boost metabolism. Test with varying meal frequency to see which works best for you and your physique's specific requirements and tastes.

Regardless of how many meals you consume per day, aim to spread them out evenly and include a variety of carbohydrates, protein, and nutritious fats to promote metabolic health and weight loss. Adhere to your own body's feeling of fullness and hunger cues, eating when your stomach growls and stopping when you're full, to maintain a positive connection with food and achieve your weight loss objectives.

4. Prior- and afterwards nutrition: nourishing your body for effectiveness and wellness.

If you're an active or frequent exerciser, paying close attention to your pre-and post-workout nutrition can make a big difference in terms of improving effectiveness, promoting recovery, and increasing fat burning. Before your physical activity, aim for a carbohydrate-protein balance to offer energy while also supporting muscle repair and growth. After exercising, restore carbohydrates and protein to replace glycogen stores, rebuild tissue in your muscles, and aid in rehab.

Practice with various pre- and post-exercise snacks and meals to see what's most effective for your body and workout schedule. Whether it's a serving of bananas and nut butter before a morning run or a nutritious protein shake after an intense strength training session, prioritize nutrient-dense foods that will help you reach your fitness objectives while keeping you energized and happy.

5. The evening Dietary requirements: Managing the Evening Hours

Ah, the evenings are a time for relaxing and unwinding after a long day, but also a time when many of us engage in mindless munching and overeating. To prevent the temptation of late-night munchies, strive to stop eating for a minimum of two to three hours before bedtime to allow for adequate digestion and avoid bloating and interrupted sleep.

If you need a snack in the evening, go for something lighter like veggies, fruits, and hummus from scratch or a small quantity of Greek yogurt to satisfy your appetite without overburdening your digestive system. Ensure to stay hydrated a glass of water or herbal tea will help you reduce your appetite and feel full till the morning of the next day.

6. Periodic Fasting: Leveraging the Benefits of Time-Restricted Eating

In the past few years, short-term fasting has become a popular dieting strategy for losing pounds and healthy metabolism, using the potency of time-restricted meals to stimulate the burning of fat while enhancing metabolism. Fasting intermittently can help balance appetite hormones, stimulate the oxidation of fat, and boost insulin response, all of which lead to increased reduction of fat and metabolic efficiency.

Explore several intermittent fasting methods to determine which works best for your body and way of life. Intermittent fasting can be a strong tool for optimizing weight and metabolic health, whether it's the 16/8 approach, in which you fast for a total of 16 hours and eat within an 8-hour glazing, or the 5:2 technique, in which you eat normally for five days and limit calories for two non-consecutive days.

Strategic eating is the conductor who plays in the big opera of losing weight and metabolic mastery, directing you on your culinary journey to maximum health and energy. Paying to concentrate on meal time, separating your snacks and meals evenly throughout the day, and prioritizing foods that are high in nutrients will help you optimize the rate of your metabolism, assist in burning calories, and uncover the path to long-term weight loss success. So, take a spoon and knife, and prepare to embark on a culinary excursion designed to nurture your body, fire up your metabolism, and boost your burning calories ability.

Cycling into Success: Exploring the Impact of Calorie cycling on Metabolism and Long-Term Weight Management

Calorie cycling is a new tactic that has entered the ever-changing field of weight control. It has the potential to completely change our understanding of diets, metabolism, and lasting results. However, what is calorie cycling exactly, and how does it operate?

Come along as we dive into the core of this cutting-edge dietary approach, learning about its effects on metabolism and how they might permanently change our outlook on how we think about managing our weight.

1. The Fundamentals of Cycling Calorie: An Exciting Adventure for Your Metabolism

Fundamentally, calorie cycling is a nutritional strategy that gradually alternates between greater and fewer calorie consumption intervals. Calorie cyclers modify their daily or weekly calorie consumption instead of adhering to a strict daily calorie target. They time their higher calorie days to correspond with periods of greater exercise or training.

The idea behind calorie cycling is straightforward: by varying the amount of calories you consume regularly, you can avoid adaptive thermogenesis, keep your metabolism guessing, and steer clear of the dreaded weight loss plateau that frequently follows conventional dieting methods. Calorie cycling essentially acts as a kind of metabolic rollercoaster, maintaining your body alert and ready to burn fat.

2. **The Science of Calorie Cycling: Creating an Effective Environment**

So is calorie cycling a genuine thing, or is it just another diet craze that will eventually go out of style? According to scientific research, calorie cycling can be a successful reduction in weight and metabolic health strategy since it can inhibit metabolic adaptation and promote long-lasting, destined fat loss.

For those who want to lose weight without compromising metabolic wellness, research has indicated that cycling between bouts of greater and lower calorie intake can prevent metabolic slowing, maintain lean muscle mass, and encourage fat loss. You may give your body the food it needs to function at its peak while also generating a calorie deficit for weight reduction by carefully scheduling your higher-calorie days to fall on times of increased exercise or training.

3. Calorie Cycling's Advantages: Beyond Just Losing Weight

Calorie cycling is an appealing diet plan for long-term success since it provides several other advantages alongside its effects on weight loss and metabolism. To begin with, calorie cycling is adaptable and flexible, letting you adjust your intake of calories to suit your unique requirements, tastes, and way of life. Calorie cycling can be customized to meet your specific needs and objectives, regardless of whether you're an athlete seeking to maximize efficiency or a busy professional managing several obligations.

Furthermore, by enabling periodic excesses without impeding your journey, calorie cycling can support the development of a positive connection with food. You may carefully incorporate days with higher calories and still lose weight by indulging in your favorite meals in balance. This flexibility and autonomy might assist avoid deprivation feelings and facilitate long-term adherence to your diet plan.

4. How to Put Calorie Cycling Into Practice: Success Strategies

Are you prepared to attempt calorie cycling? Here are some pointers to help you put this novel food plan into practice and increase the likelihood of success:

To begin, determine your baseline energy requirements by speaking with a trained nutritionist or utilizing a reliable internet calculator.

- Once you know your baseline caloric goal, try out several cycling programmes to see which suits you the best. While certain individuals prefer to shift between days with greater and lower calories within a single week, others prefer to change their calorie intake on a weekly schedule.

Think about including foods that are rich in nutrients that assist prolonged energy, wellness, and performance when organizing your higher-calorie days. When it comes to making sure you're getting enough nutrients, try to strike a balance between protein, carbs, and healthy fats.

Pay attention to your body's signals of hunger and fullness and be cautious of portion amounts. Even if you can enjoy days with higher calories, it's crucial to avoid going overboard and undoing the calorie deficit you've established on days with lower calories.

Keep a close eye on your development and adapt as necessary. If you're not getting the desired results, think about adjusting your calorie cycling regimen or seeking individualized advice from a specialist.

5. The Possible Consequences of Calorie Cycling: Things to Remember

Calorie cycling has some potential disadvantages even though it can be a useful weight loss and metabolic condition therapy. Calorie cycling's intrinsic flexibility and freedom may cause overeating or binge eating in certain individuals, especially on days when their daily caloric intake is higher. Furthermore, not every individual can benefit from calorie cycling, particularly those with a track record of eating disorders or specific medical issues.

It's also important to remember that calorie cycling is not always successful and that it takes meticulous preparation and care to detail. The advantages of the cycle strategy may be defeated if inadequate measuring and tracking make it simple to overeat on days when you should be eating more calories or unintentionally build an excess of calories.

Lastly, it's critical to keep in mind that calorie cycling is only one weight control strategy in the arsenal. Though it's not a panacea and isn't likely to yield big effects by itself, it can be a useful tactic for certain people. Calorie cycling works best when combined with other good lifestyle practices that promote general well-being, such as regular exercise, getting adequate rest, and managing pressure.

Calorie cycling is a potential new strategy that leverages precise timing to maximize metabolism, boost fat loss, and foster steady progress in the larger weight management puzzle. You may prevent adaptive thermogenesis, keep your metabolism guessing, and avoid the much-discussed weight loss barrier that frequently follows standard dieting methods by cycling between periods of greater and lower calorie intake. So fasten your seatbelts and get yourself ready for an exhilarating journey into the realm of calorie cycling, where achievement is but a few cycles ahead.

Chapter 4

Enhancing Metabolic health with Functional Foods: Harnessing the power of functional foods to boost metabolism, support fat loss, and improve overall health.

In the busy world of nutrition, a new category of superfoods has emerged, a group of potent companions known as productive foods, each possessing the capacity to nourish your body, increase your metabolism, and improve your wellness from the inside out. But what exactly are functional meals, and how can they assist optimize metabolic health, support weight loss, and improve overall wellness? Join us as we go on a trip into the realm of healthy foods, discovering their unique features and learning the secrets of nature's medicine to optimize metabolism and alter your health.

1. The Power of Functional Foods: Nature's Pharmacy

At their heart, functional foods are full, nutritious foods that go beyond simply providing basic nutrition to give additional health advantages beyond their essential components. From rich in antioxidants to berries to omega-3-packed oily fish, these nutritional foods are a natural pharmacy, a golden wealth of active substances that can boost metabolic health, improve immunity, and reduce the likelihood of chronic illnesses.

Unlike old-fashioned processed food items, which may be stripped of their vital nutrients and loaded with chemical additives, functional foods are less processed and wrapped with a wide array of nutrients, minerals, antioxidants, and phytonutrients that work together to enable ideal well-being and longevity.

2. **Utilizing the Healing Effects of Plant-based Nutrients: Plant-Powered Medicine**

At the heart of many functional foods lies a group of potent molecules that are called phytonutrients bioactive substances found in plants that exhibit unique health-promoting qualities. From the striking colors of vegetables and fruits to the pungent odors of herbs and spices, antioxidants are the secret equipment of nature's pharmacy, each giving a distinct set of advantages for metabolic health and general wellness.

For example, polyphenols present in foods like berries, leafy green tea, and dark-coloured chocolate have been scientifically demonstrated to boost heart health, decrease inflammation, and enhance the breakdown of fat. Similarly, carotenoids present in foods like carrots, which are sweet potatoes, and green leafy veggies have been attributed to increased vision, enhanced immune function, and lower risk for long-lasting ailments.

3. Promoting a Healthy Gut with Bacteria and Prebiotics or Developing Healthy microbes

Besides their role in delivering critical nutrients and antioxidants, functional foods also play a key role in maintaining gut health, an often-overlooked facet of metabolic health and general wellness. The gut of my microbiome, comprising billions of bacteria alongside other microorganisms, plays a key role in digestion, nutrition absorption, immunological function, and metabolism.

By adding nutritious foods high in probiotics and beneficial bacteria which encourage gut health such as milk products, kefir, cabbage, and kimchi, you may assist with building a robust microbiome that aids proper digestion and metabolism. In a comparable manner foods high in prebiotic indigestible fibers that serve as energy for helpful gut microorganisms such as garlic, onions, leeks, and bananas, may help replenish your gut flora and support a balanced proportion of friendly microbes.

4. **Maintaining Blood Sugar with Fiber and amino acids: regulating Optimal Energy and Minimising Food cravings**

When it comes to metabolic wellness, glucose management is crucial. Spikes and dips in the blood sugar level may cause damage to the body's metabolism, triggering exhaustion, hunger pangs, and gaining weight. Well, panic and non-functional foods are here to ease your worries.

By integrating foods high in proteins and fibers into your diet such as whole grains, legumes, lentils, nuts, seeds, and lean meats you may help balance blood sugar levels, minimize energy dumps, and keep cravings at bay. Fiber slows the breakdown of sugars into the circulatory system, while protein helps regulate appetite hormones and increase feelings of fullness, resulting in important friends in the fight over metabolic disorders.

5. Increasing Metabolism with Thermogenic Foods: Turning Up the Heat on Fat Burning

If you're trying to fire up your metabolism and boost fat burning, look no further than thermostatic meals that raise the body's calorie-burning capability by increasing central temperature and raising the rate of digestion.

Hot meals like hot peppers, cayenne pepper, and ginger include chemicals like capsaicin and gingerol, which have been demonstrated to boost thermogenesis and stimulate the breakdown of fat. Similarly, caffeine-containing meals including coffee, herbal tea, and dark chocolate can stimulate the central nervous system and increase the rate of metabolism, resulting in more calories burned and improved fat reduction.

Incorporating Functional Foods into Your Diet: Tips for Success

Ready to take advantage of the power of nutritious foods and boost your overall health? Here are some strategies for adding these formidable companions into your diet and receiving the advantages of the natural world's medicine:

Fill your plate with a rainbow of energetic fruits and veggies, aiming for a diversity of hues to guarantee you're getting a diverse array of vitamins, minerals, and antioxidants.

Incorporate lean proteins like fish, meat, poultry, tofu, and lentils into the food you eat and snack on to facilitate muscular development and repair, regulate hunger hormones, and boost feelings of fullness.

Add herbs and spices like spice turmeric, cinnamon, which is and garlic to the food you prepare to increase flavor and add a hefty dose of phytonutrients along with antioxidants to your meals.

Explore foods that ferment like yogurt, kefir, sour cabbage and kimchi (fermented cabbage) to improve gut health and foster an established microbiome.

Be mindful that healthy fats incorporate nutrients like avocado, nuts, seeds, and oil from olives into your diet to boost brain function, hormone production, and nutrient absorption.

In the epic orchestral work of nutrition, nutritious foods stand as the virtuosos of nature's healthcare, each having the power to fuel your body, improve your metabolism, and modify your well-being from the inside out. By leveraging the medicinal benefits of the phytonutrients promoting gut health, regulating blood sugar levels, and introducing thermogenic foods into your diet, you can improve your metabolic health, promote fat reduction, and discover the key to robust health and energy. So, fill your stomach with nature's greatest offerings, and become ready to take care of your physical being, boost your metabolism, and flourish like rarely in the past.

Identifying key superfoods and their specific benefits for metabolic function and longevity.

In the broad realm of nutrition, there are particular foods which stand out as proven superheroes. These meals are loaded with powerful nutrients and chemicals that can improve metabolic function, encourage fat loss, and boost longevity. Take part in us as we embark on a trip into the globe in search of these nutrient-rich powerhouses, where we will discover the unique health advantages that these foods offer for metabolic function and longevity, as well as the keys to robust wellness and energy.

2. Berries, in particular, are known as the antioxidant powerhouses of nature

Berries, which are overflowing with brilliant colors and sweet flavors, are a blessing from nature to our taste buds as well as to our digestive system. The antioxidant-rich raspberries and fruit like strawberries, in addition to exotic superfruits like acai fruits and goji berries, are just two examples of the powerful substances that can be found in these bite-sized jewels. These compounds have the potential to improve metabolic efficiency, aid in fat loss, and increase longevity.

Berries, which are abundant in polyphenols such as cyan pigments, compounds called flavonoids and vitamin C, support the neutralization of free radicals, the reduction of inflammatory conditions, and the protection against oxidative stress, which is a significant factor in the development of chronic diseases and the aging process. Furthermore, the high fiber found in berries tends to facilitate fullness, the regulation of glucose levels in the blood, and the aid of digestive health, which makes them an invaluable collaborator in the pursuit of metabolic longevity and optimal health.

2. Oily seafood is a nutritional superstar that is rich in omega-3 fatty acids.

Fish such as salmon, sardines, and mackerel are examples of fatty seafood that perform exceptionally well when it comes to extending lifespan and maintaining the function of the metabolic system. Packed with omega-3 fatty acids EPA as well as DHA, these watery heroines assist in reducing inflammatory processes, lower levels of triglycerides, and improve heart health a critical component of overall life.

It has also been demonstrated that fatty acids known as omega-3 promote metabolic function by increasing sensitivity to insulin, decreasing swelling in fat cells, and encouraging fat oxidation. As a result, they are an excellent supplement for any diet that is centered on controlling the accumulation of weight and the maintenance of metabolic health. Aim to integrate oily fish into your diet at least twice per week to receive the full advantages of these omega-3 fatty acids power stations.

3. Leafy Greens: Rich in nutrients Partners for Metabolism Knowledge

the cartoon character Popeye was onto something when he went for a can of greens to power his incredible strength. Green leafy vegetables like cabbage, kale, spinach, and Swiss chard are nutrient-rich powerhouses, rich with nutrients such as vitamins, minerals and phytochemicals that improve the efficiency of the metabolism, stimulate fat loss, and boost overall health and vigor.

Rich in the antioxidants vitamins A, C, and K, as well as folic acid, potassium, and the mineral magnesium, leafy greens help maintain metabolism in cells, control glucose levels in the blood, and defend against oxidative stress a threefold danger against metabolic malfunction and chronic disease. Furthermore, the substantial amount of fiber in green vegetables helps increase feeling full, control absorption, and promote healthy weight, making them an invaluable tool in the search for metabolic processes mastery.

4. The ingredient turmeric: The Golden Flavour for Sustainability

For generations, spice turmeric has been valued for its medical characteristics and medicinal properties. Loaded with curcumin, another potent antioxidant and soothing component, turmeric has been demonstrated to boost metabolic activity, reduce inflammatory processes, and increase lifespan.

Green tea: A panacea of long-term sustainability and a metabolic booster Green tea, which has been consumed for millennia in traditional Asian civilizations, is more than simply a calming drink; it also functions as a lifespan potion and a metabolic stimulant. Rich in catechins, a powerful class of antioxidant compounds, green tea is an antioxidant that supports weight loss, improves metabolic efficiency, and enhances general health and vigor.

Catechins have been scientifically demonstrated to enhance insulin sensitivity, decrease inflammatory processes, and encourage fat oxidation in addition to increasing the process of thermogenesis or the body's ability to burn calories.

This is a potent combination for maintaining a healthy metabolism and controlling weight. To fully enjoy the metabolic advantages of green tea, replace your midday coffee with a cup of this superfood.

These nutritional powerhouses are real heroes in the grand scheme of dietary intake, full of powerful nutrients and chemicals that can boost the lifespan, improve the rate of metabolism, and encourage fat loss. These powerhouses of nutrition offer a wealth of advantages for anyone looking to maximize their health and vitality, from metabolism-boosting spices like spice turmeric and green tea to rich-in nutrients greens such as spinach and omega-3-rich fatty fish. So load up on the best that nature has to provide and get ready to discover the keys to mastering metabolism and living a long life.

Chapter 5

Exercises and Movement for Metabolic Mastery

Incorporating exercise and physical activity into your routine to enhance metabolism, burn fat, and improve metabolic health.

In a constantly changing movement of metabolic power, movement and physical activity take center stage, providing a potent tool for increasing metabolism, burning fat, and improving metabolism in general. This chapter looks into the transforming power of vigorous physical activity, showing how integrating fitness into your daily routine could open the door to metabolic power and vigor.

1. The Power of Activity Boosting Your Metabolic Fire.

Movement is medicine, a powerful potion that may fire up your metabolic combustion chamber, increase fat burning, and boost your energy levels. From vigorous strolls and strength training exercises to yoga courses and dance training sessions, every activity you do has the potential to boost your metabolism while enhancing your metabolic condition.

Being active not only consumes calories and develops muscle, but it also helps manage the level of blood sugar, enhance insulin sensitivity, and reduce inflammation, all of which benefit the metabolic process and general health. By including consistent physical activity in your routine, you may use the power of movement to boost your body's metabolism and alter your state of mind from within.

2. **Resistance Exercise for Metabolic Muscle**

When it involves boosting your metabolism and reducing body fat, exercise with weights is your hidden weapon. Resistance exercises such as lunges, and performing deadlifts can help you gain lean muscle mass, increase the speed of your metabolism, and improve insulin sensitivity all of which are beneficial for regulating your metabolism.

In contrast to constant state cardio, which burns calories primarily during activity, strength training has a metabolic afterburn effect known as excess after an activity consumption of oxygen (EPOC), which maintains calories even after your workout is completed. Furthermore, exercising with weights helps to maintain healthy muscle mass throughout the loss of weight, minimizing metabolic slowdown and encouraging long-term fat loss effectiveness.

3. Heart and circulatory Exercise: Boosting Fat Burn

While strength training is important for muscle growth and metabolism, aerobic activity is critical for increasing fat-burning and enhancing cardiovascular health. Aerobic exercise, whether you're jogging, strolling, swimming, or swaying, raises your heart rate, burns more calories, and improves aerobic capacity, a triple threat to metabolic imbalance and persistent illness.

Cardiovascular fitness also improves insulin sensitivity, reduces inflammatory processes, and promotes fat burning, making it a crucial part of any metabolic-focused exercise plan. To maximize the metabolic condition advantages of cardiovascular fitness, aim for at least 160 minutes of aerobics with moderate intensity or 70 minutes of high-intensity aerobic activity per week.

4. Mentally and physically Practices for Harmonising Mind and Soul

Apart from weight training and aerobic exercise, mind-body practices such as yoga, tai chi, and qigong provide an integrated path to metabolic mastery by integrating movement and mindfulness to nourish your entire being. These modest but effective activities assist in minimizing tension, increasing the quality of sleep, and boosting general well-being, all of which are necessary for good metabolic function.

Integrating mental and physical exercises into your routine allows you to tap into the fundamental connection between your mind and body, reduce your level of cortisol, and produce a state of calm and balance which fosters metabolic optimal functioning. Whether you're doing a sun salutation or finding quiet in a meditation practice, mind-body practices can help boost metabolism while enhancing your general health.

In the entire work. metabolism mastery, movement and physical activity provide the crescendo of tremendous climax that fires your metabolic fire, melts fat, and enhances your general wellness and energy. By adding exercise for strength, cardiovascular workouts, and mental-body exercises into your daily schedule, you can capitalize on the transforming power of exercise to boost the rate of your metabolism, improve your health, and uncover the way to long-term vitality. So, buckle up your trainers, spread out the yoga floor and prepare to move your path to metabolic mastery over them.

Exploring Different Types of Exercise and Their Effects on Metabolism

In the rich pattern of metabolic processes mastery, durability is the precious thread that sutures together routines and conducts into a fabric of sustainable wellness and enthusiasm. To embark on the final part of this journey, let's delve into the art of creating sustainable techniques for permanent success, nurturing behaviors which promote an efficient metabolism and maintain a reduction in weight for an extended period.

The Road Ahead Begins: A Personalized Analysis

Let me accompany you on an exploration through my personal experience, a trip defined by ups and downs and the discovery of the transformational effect of sustainable routines. Like many,

I've experienced the hurdles of weight reduction and metabolic well-being, traveling through fad diets, fast cures, and periods of discouragement. But it had been via failures and successes, and an attitude of dedication to long-lasting improvement, that I uncovered my road to permanent achievement.

The Basis of Long-term Sustainability: Little Processes, Vast Effect

At the center of lasting success lies the realization that small actions can result in major progress. Rather than pursuing drastic modifications that are untenable in years to come, concentrate on creating modest, manageable improvements to your way of life. Start by implementing one beneficial habit at a time, whether it's adding a portion of veggies to your diet, engaging in an everyday walk, or adopting conscious eating and enabling these tiny adjustments to aggregate gradually, providing a firm basis for permanent success.

The Power of Awareness Nutrition: Rich in nutrients Body and Soul

A mindful diet is far more than just a trend; it's an effective discipline that may improve your connection with meals and support metabolic health over time. By listening to your body's satiety and fullness signals, exercising portion control, and savoring each mouthful, you may build a conscious approach to eating that fosters stability, contentment, and lasting control of weight. Keep in mind it's not solely the foods you eat, but how you eat that's essential.

Discovering Pleasure in Activity Recognising the Therapeutic Benefits of Workout

Workout is typically perceived as a chore, but it doesn't necessarily need to be. Instead of pushing oneself to struggle through workouts you detest, find joy in exercise by investigating hobbies that offer you happiness and fulfillment. Whether it's performing arts, biking, swimming, or doing yoga, the goal is to discover hobbies that you enjoy that also fit perfectly into your routine. By adopting exercise as an expression of joy and vitality, you'll be more

inclined to remain with it for a long time, earning metabolic advantages along the way.

Establishing a Positive Space: encircling Yourself with Positivity

They say that your self-worth is the average of the five individuals whom you utilize most of your moments with, so why don't you encircle yourself with a positive value and aid in it? Whether it's attending a gym session, checking out other like-minded individuals via the internet, or soliciting the assistance of a relative or close friend, developing an effective network of support can make all possible progress on your route to long-term success. Surround yourself with individuals who inspire and motivate you, and who share your dedication to living a healthy, vibrant life.

Embracing Flexibility: Adapting to Life's Ups and Downs

Reality is unpredictable, and remaining on a path with your fitness goals can be tough amid unforeseen setbacks and hurdles. That's why it's crucial to embrace flexibility and adaptability, realizing that growth is never entirely smooth. Instead of perceiving setbacks as failures, see them as chances for growth and learning. Be nice to yourself, exercise self-care, and realize that each passing day is an opportunity to begin new and to adhere to your objectives.

Embracing Growth, Without Flawlessness: Appreciating Your Path

In the quest for sustained achievement, it's crucial to appreciate progress, not flawlessness. Understand that effective change requires time and effort and that each action you take heading towards a better, healthier life is a win deserving of recognition. if it's fitting into a favorite pair of pants you haven't put on in years, learning a new yoga posture, or just feeling refreshed and alive, take the moment to appreciate and enjoy your victories along your path.

The Road Trip Continues: A Lifetime of Wellness and Vitality

As we approach the closing of this section, let us recall that the path to metabolism control is not their final destination, but a lifetime effort. By building sustainable lifestyles and actions, nurturing our physical bodies and minds, and adopting the power of tiny, relentless improvements, we can establish a solid basis for permanent energy and well-being that will take us through a lifetime of well-being. So, let us commence on this path together, helping and motivating each other

as we seek to live our most
fulfilling lives full of energy, life,
and pleasure.

Chapter 6

Sustainable Strategies for Long-Term Success

Allow me to impart an individual tale as we wrap up the chapter on metabolic control. I've experienced both highs and lows while trying to lose weight, like many others have. But what made a difference was realizing that long-term behaviors were more important than band-aid solutions. I found that making tiny, regular adjustments like switching from processed to whole foods as munchies and discovering the joy of movement produced long-lasting effects. Thus, I'm inviting you to adopt an equivalent viewpoint. Let's work together to build enduring habits that will nourish the cells in our bodies, uplift our spirits, and set us on the path to eternal vitality and optimal health.

Making a Plan for Optimal Nutrition and Energy Throughout Life

Starting a path towards long-term health and vitality necessitates having a roadmap, a strategy that helps you overcome roadblocks, maintains your motivation, and gives you the ability to persevere through difficulties regardless of what.

1. **Establish Measurable Objectives**: Establish attainable objectives that are consistent with your vision for health and vitality first. Whether your goal is to run an entire marathon, lose a specific amount of weight, or just feel more alive and energetic, having a unique feeling of purpose can help

you remain focused and inspired along the way.

2. **Split It Right:** Divide your objectives into more doable, smaller tasks that you can complete one at a time. By concentrating on manageable accomplishments, you'll gain trust and determination as you get closer to your bigger goals.

3. **Remain Adaptable:** Difficulties will inevitably come since life is

unpredictable. Remain adaptive and fluid, and be ready to modify your strategy as necessary. Consider obstacles as chances for advancement and growth rather than as shortcomings.

4. Identify Your Support Network: Embrace a network of friends, family, or fellow wellness enthusiasts who will strive to promote you when you crave it most. Having a solid support

network can be crucial for maintaining motivation and getting beyond challenges.

5. **Show off Your Improvement**: Regardless of how minor your accomplishments may seem, give them some thought. Celebrate your accomplishments and recognise how far you've reached on your path to health and vitality, whether it's hitting a goal, learning a new skill, or just staying true to

what you have planned for another day of success.

6. **Continue to remain Motivated**: Look for ideas that speak to you to stay driven and inspired. Discover methods to stay inspired to keep pushing forward by staying connected to your vision through activities such as studying literature, catching up on podcasts, or audio or watching

social media accounts which give positive messages and ideas.

You may confidently, resolutely, and determinedly handle the ups and downs of your health path by making a plan for lifetime health and vitality and using techniques for conquering setbacks and maintaining motivation. With an awareness of goal and dedication, put on your trainers, take your bottle of water, and set off on the path towards good health and vitality, believing that each step will be worthwhile in the process.

Conclusion

Finally, "Strategize Meals to Boost Your Diet and Health" provides an in-depth analysis of achieving peak health through strategic meal planning. This book emphasizes the importance of diet, giving readers the tools they need to lose excess calories, live a healthier and fitter lifestyle, lengthen their lives, and naturally enhance their metabolism.

Readers may revolutionize their eating habits by combining intelligent advice with practical ideas, paving the path for long-term success in weight control and overall well-being.

This book emphasizes the significance of proportion and various kinds in meal planning. Instead of severe diets or rigid eating habits, the author recommends a more sustainable strategy that emphasizes including a varied range of nutrient-dense foods in one's diet. Individuals can meet their dietary requirements while enjoying an array of vegetables, fruits, whole grains, lean proteins, and healthy fats.

Beyond that, the book emphasizes the need for mindful eating for general health and wellness. Giving attention to hunger signals, adopting portion management, and savoring each bite can help people create a healthier connection with food and avoid overeating. Furthermore, the book urges readers to be careful of their food choices, preferring whole, unprocessed foods whenever feasible and avoiding overly processed, nutrient-poor alternatives.

Another significant attribute of the book is its emphasis on meal timing and frequency. Rather than sticking to tight meal plans, the author advises readers to pay closer attention to their bodies and have meals when hungry. Individuals who space their meals evenly throughout the day and include nutritious snacks as needed can maintain consistent energy levels and avoid the pitfalls of severe hunger or overeating.

Furthermore, the book provides vital information about the importance of water in overall health and well-being. Individuals who stay hydrated throughout the day can assist their metabolism, maintain gut health, and increase overall energy levels. The author suggests drinking plenty of water and including hydrating items like veggies and fruit in snacks as meals.

In addition, "Strategize Meals to Boost Your Diet and Health" emphasizes the value of regular physical activity alongside a nutritious diet. Individuals who incorporate a combination of aerobic exercise, strength training, and flexibility exercises into their routines can maximize their weight reduction efforts, improve overall fitness levels, and improve metabolic function.

In addition to practical guidance on meal planning and vigorous physical activity, the book discusses the role of mentality and motivation in reaching long-term health objectives. Individuals can overcome challenges and stay on course for success by establishing achievable goals, adhering to healthy behaviors, and seeking assistance from friends, family, or a healthcare professional.

Ultimately, "Strategize Meals to Boost balance Diet and Health" is an excellent resource for anyone trying to improve their eating habits, enhance their health, or meet their weight loss objectives. By emphasizing the significance of balance, diversity, and mindful eating, the book enables readers to take control of their health and achieve long-term changes. This book offers practical recommendations, insightful counsel, and proven strategies for reaching maximum wellness and good health.